Good Health and Long Life is possible if you can work towards achieving it!

HOW TO ACHIEVE GOOD HEALTH AND LONG LIFE

By

Clement O. Ofiemo

DEDICATION

This book is dedicated to Almighty God who made it possible for this book to become a reality. I give special thanks to God for giving me the time, strength and wisdom to write and make this book available to all those who are serious and interested in achieving good health and long life; may God inspire people to read this book and for them to realize that good health and long life is attainable by not only praying to God but also that everyone has a responsibility and a role to play in bringing about good health and long life.

ACKNOWLEDGEMENT

I wish to acknowledge and give special thanks to all those who contributed directly or indirectly in the production of this book. May God Almighty bless you all with good health and long life.

PREFACE

Achieving good health and long life is a subject which many people take for granted. Many people just assume that good health will always manifest for them if they just believe in God and pray earnestly for good health; most people just think God will give them good health without consciously making
any real effort to achieving it.

I have often wondered why people just imagine that God will do everything for them without taking some responsibility. So many people live anyhow and eat just anything they like without knowing that they need to avoid certain food, drinks and other consumables items that can jeopardize their health.

I think there is a real need for some level of enlightenment to be given to the general public to raise the level of awareness for people to be actively involved in securing their health. I have deliberately summarized the content of this book so as to make it brief and easily readable considering the fact that many people don't seem to have enough time to read bulky books in these days of internet browsing and television watching. This book will go a long way in guiding and providing valuable hints or tips for those who really care about good health and long life.

TABLE OF CONTENTS

GOOD HEALTH

Life will certainly be more meaningful if we can enjoy it with little or no stress and even much better if we can enjoy it without any health challenges at all. Living a life of good health is not only a possibility but it is also a reality since many people with the right knowledge of what to do to achieve good health have already started enjoying good vibrant health up till their old age and even till their very last breath, in many parts of the world.

Living a happy life without the discomfort that goes with many of the health challenges we face today is not a difficult thing to achieve if we are really serious about achieving it. It only requires the will and discipline to bring it about, and so many people have been able to demonstrate this reality already, so I strongly believe that if they can achieve it, then you too can do the same.

Achieving good health is not rocket science; achieving good health and long life is not as expensive as previously believed. A little monetary investment might be necessary at the initial stage of preparing to kick start the journey of good health and long life but I strongly believe that it is very well worth it as no amount of money is comparable or equal in value to a human life. A human life cannot be compared or quantified in monetary terms. Many people save a lot of money or even acquire loans to buy things like landed properties, cars, cloths, shoes and other things to enable them enjoy life and feel good but it seems so many people are not so willing to save money or borrow (loan) money to acquire what they really need to maintain or achieve good health and long life. Many people think more about acquiring material things of life without really thinking of how to preserve their precious lives which is what will enable them to remain alive to enjoy these material things. But of what use is earthly or worldly possessions if you will not be alive or healthy enough to enjoy them?

The principle of self preservation is the first law of life. Self preservation is the primary responsibility of everyone. Anyone who does not care about good health can best be described as a "reckless" individual. We did not create ourselves and life should be seen as a gift of the creator to us and this gift should not be treated as a worthless gift. Anyone who does not value his or her life may end up losing it much quicker than those people who value their lives and are doing everything humanly possible to preserve it. Even the animals do struggle or fight in the face of danger to preserve themselves to remain alive when threatened, not to talk of a more intelligent creature like "MAN".

Life is meant to be lived and enjoyed for the benefit of man and to the glory of God. Therefore everything humanly possible should always be done to preserve one's life and to always keep it in a very good healthy state. Preserving life should therefore not only be limited to preserving only our own life but also to the preservation of the lives of others since we all need one another to exist side by side to make live meaningful. If most people around us are sick or unhealthy, we can be affected one way or another. The sick person might be the one you need to provide you some essential goods or services and this might not be possible since he or she is now sick when you need the service. If you are well and other members of your family are sick, the burden of their sickness will directly affect you too, you will certainly be affected one way or another; it may cost you some money to help in their treatment or even prevent you from doing other things since you will be compelled to spend some of your valuable time caring for them.

Even in your place of work the absence of a key member (or some members) of staff from duty as a result of sickness will disrupt business activities and this might create some form of inconveniences to other staff members as they may have to adjust themselves to perform the duties of those absent staff members until they are fit enough to return back to work or the work of the absent members of staff is simply left undone until they return and this may affect the organization in many ways. Which ever way you look at it, sickness or ill health will definitely affect us one way or another whether we are the ones who are sick or anybody else. Sickness can be very risky if not tamed and banished from our lives. It may cost you your job and source of income, it may lead to a sack if you are always sick, because your employer may sack you for being always absent from duty as no one will like to employ or keep an employee who is always sick. It is therefore our responsibility to always do everything within our powers to protect or preserve our health and to prevent any situation that can change our state of good health to a state of ill health or sickness of any kind. Allowing sickness or diseases to strike us can be too risk because not everyone is always lucky enough to escape with their lives; some people might be lucky to escape with some damages or disabilities but some others may unfortunately end up in their graves.

Some sickness or diseases are some how unavoidable but I think it is totally unacceptable for anyone to lose his or her life as a result of any sickness or disease which can be avoided or prevented; dying from a disease or sickness which can be prevented or within the absolute control of a victim is to suffer what I call "AVOIDABLE DEATH"; suffering an impairment or disability due to an avoidable health problem is suffering an "AVOIDABLE DISABILITY".

HEALTH CHALLENGES

As someone who has experienced the devastating conditions that can arise from being sick, I have taken a very keen interest in not only attaining good health but also how to remain permanently in a constant state of health. I have taken my time to do some research of how to attain good health over the years and at some point in time was considering the possibility of going back to school to study "medicine" or a related discipline or course, but after taking a look at some other factors I was discouraged from embarking on any cause of action. One thing that initially held me back was what I perceive as the lackadaisical attitude of many health workers and the unreliable system of health care that is increasingly falling to provide or meet the health needs of the people in many cases. Many health workers don't seem to know exactly why they have been employed or many of them are simply not interested in the health care aspect of the job while showing so much interest in the money or the wealth they can get out of the health care system. Some of these health workers are so uncaring to the extent of either deliberately ignoring the patients or always exhibiting rude behaviors that can sometimes put their patients off. Some of these health workers will prefer to refer or direct you to other hospitals (especially to hospitals owned by them or their associates) to seek medical care or treatment; they are more interested in how much money they can make from the patients and not their well being.

I have been to the government owned "General Hospitals" in Nigeria and have seen the multitude of people who throng there to seek medical help. Sometimes the crowd is so much that they virtually overwhelm the health workers working in those hospitals. Apart from the fact that some of these health workers, nurses, doctors and others are not really people with selfless disposition who are willing to render selfless service to their fellow humans with compassion without seeking for a reward in return, sometimes the sheer number of patients seeking medical help can be so much and enough to frustrate or over stress even the most dedicated health worker and make him or her unwilling to continue to render medical help beyond a particular tolerance limit.

I am very thankful and very grateful to God that I have never been sick and still pray that I will never be sick up to the extent of being admitted in a hospital bed to sleep overnight or spend some nights in any of the "General Hospitals" in Nigeria, though I believe that I personally will never be sick again to be admitted to any hospital anywhere, I detest sickness and I believe that by the grace of God all sickness is forever banished from my life. But I have spent some nights in some "General Hospitals" where I have the responsibility to provide some extra care for a loved one (some of these hospital will actually demand that a family member of a patient should spend the night to help provide some form of support to the sick person), I must admit here that the experience of spending some nights in these "General Hospitals" was not a pleasant experience. Apart from the extremely poor sanitary conditions of these hospitals, the necessary things needed to make the general environment conducive within and outside the wards or residential quarters are inadequate or non existent. The presence of flies, mosquitoes and other insects in some of these hospitals is no doubts a threat not only to the patients but also to the people who are not sick but have been compelled to stay there to help provide some form of care to their loved ones. Spending some nights in some of these hospital can be a real nightmare whether you are sick or not sick; I as a person do not cherish the idea of spending even a night in such places not to talk about staying in such places over some weeks like some people do because of either being sick or being there to provide extra care to their loved ones.

I have on few occasions seen people suffer helplessly in some hospitals not only due to neglect by the medical workers but also due to the fact that the medical personnel's are unable to provide an effective treatment, remedy or medical help due to the fact that they have done their very best based on the knowledge at their disposal and there is nothing else that they can do to help the patients since the patients medical case is beyond their capacity or has simply defied medical treatments. I remember a particular case of a pregnant woman who was in critical labour pains. She cried and begged for whatever medical help throughout the night in one "General Hospital" where I happened to have spent one night in a typical Nigerian hospital, to stay with my loved one who was there to "Give Birth" or "Deliver a Child". This woman's case was very pathetic because she was in extreme pains and was just shouting for help non stop throughout the night. I heard the medical personnel's saying some words of comfort and after a while she was just left alone until the doctor arrived. After examining the pregnant woman, I heard the doctor saying she should get everything ready for a "caesarian section operation" and was told to pay some huge amount of money which further alarmed the already distressed pregnant woman. I could hear her pleading with the doctor to help her out since she does not have the money demanded by the medical personnel for the "caesarian section operation". The doctor only sympathized with the woman and calmly explained to the woman that there is nothing else he can do without the money for the operation and left the scene. The wailing and weeping of the pregnant woman continued. She just kept on crying, crying and asking for whatever help possible. This incident happened in the night between the hours of, if I can still remember correctly around 11.00 pm to 5.00 am. I happened to travel to this hospital from a near by village to see my wife who was also there to deliver a baby, she was referred to this hospital from the other hospital in the village where I was working then, my wife was referred there because according to the nurses her case was beyond their help as she has been in labour pains for sometime without being able to deliver her baby so she was rushed in a motorcycle to this hospital for a possible "caesarian section operation". They said the doctor was not on sit and that even if he was on sit that in the event of an operation they do not have the facility to carryout a "caesarian section operation".

The use of cell phones was not in vogue then so I did not know that my wife has been rushed to this hospital because I travelled to this same town where the hospital is located in the morning to buy some necessary baby things after taking my wife to the other hospital where we live so when I returned from the town, I went straight to the village hospital only to be told that my wife has been rushed to the other hospital in the town in a motorcycle since vehicles don't usually ply our roads due to the very deplorable state of the road at that time. I immediately returned back to the town hospital and by the time I got there it was too late to come back home so I had to plead with some hospital staff to let me sleep somewhere in the hospital (they provided a nearby empty room for me to sleep). I tried to sleep but I could not, so I just lay on the bed. Luckily and happily for me my wife delivered our baby in what I will describe as the first miracle because I thought that my wife was going to undergo a "caesarean operation" because that was why they referred us to this hospital but as it turned out my wife delivered safely without a "caesarean operation".

This heavily pregnant woman who could not deliver her baby was still crying for help when the doctor left her as a result of her inability to pay the money demanded for the "caesarean operation". I was highly touched. I could not sleep so I remembered what I read sometime ago in a book titled: "You Too Can Heal" written by His Eminence Sir George King, the Metropolitan Archbishop of the Aetherius Churches. In this book the Archbishop gave some healing tips about how to give spiritual healing to anyone in distress or sick. So I rose from where I was lying and I decided to just try this healing ideology hoping that it might help this woman in her state of distress. I started praying and directing prayer energy as taught by the Archbishop to the direction of where I guess this woman might be according to the sound of her cries. I prayed earnestly but silently as much as I could, wishing this woman a miracle of safe delivery; I was asking God to intervene and make it possible for the woman to give birth to her child without any further pains or problem and I stated quite strongly that she will deliver without any "caesarean operation." I prayed and chanted a "healing mantra" as instructed by the writer of that book for quite sometime and after a while I noticed that the woman became a bit calm; her cries for help reduced drastically and I gradually started relaxing my prayers until I decided to stop. I decided to lay down and before I knew it I slept off.

As soon as I woke up the next morning, I decided to go into the delivery ward to see my wife and I asked about what happened to the woman who was crying all night due to her inability to deliver, only to discover that another miracle had happened while I was fast asleep. The woman had delivered safely without any complication or "caesarean operation." I just smiled and walk straight to where the woman and her baby was lying down and greeted them and thanking God for her safe delivery. I realized that it was unnecessary to say a word about my prayers for her and I just walked away feeling good. I had no doubt in my mind that God had just done another miracle through the little effort of an unholy man. When I reflected upon the statement made by the writer of the book "You Too Can Heal" that it is the birthright of everybody to give healing because everyone can do it if the right knowledge of how to give healing is properly learned and practiced, I realized that he was right. I have on some other occasion followed the counsel of this healing book and found it very effective.

I have on many occasions heard of women who went to the hospital to give birth to their baby but were unable to do so successfully for one reason or the other. I have heard of very complicated child births or deliveries that either led to the death of the women or the baby concerned or both of them dying in the process. In some cases the women had to undergo "caesarian operation" before the baby could be delivered. One of the reasons why I started showing interest in finding a possible solution to this child delivery problem was because it is becoming very rampant or common. It is gradually becoming a norm that these days that if about ten women goes to the hospital for child delivery there is no guarantee that all of them will be able deliver their baby safely without some of them getting assistance through "caesarian operation". This is a very delicate situation and I think it is not normal. In those days, this kind of thing was almost non existent; it was almost unheard of that a woman went to give birth to her baby and came back home without the baby or even didn't come back alive; it was very rare. People are not so sure what will happen now when a woman goes to the hospital for child birth; in many cases now, every family member is highly tensed up when a woman enters a labour room these days to give birth to a baby. This should not be so. Although some people believe that this situation can be caused by spiritual attack (especially in

Africa) but even if it is so in some cases, I don't think it is true in many cases.

The good news is that, due to some serious research by experienced medical scientists a very reliable solution has been found to help solve this problem or at least reduce this problem of difficult child birth to the barest minimum. Many of the health practices briefly discussed in this book has a direct bearing on some of the solution so far propounded to help solve this problem. Since the purpose of writing this book is not to advertise or sell any medication or health products to anyone, I will not be able to go into details by mentioning some very good prescription but suffice to say that there are some strict health practices to be followed and some very good natural health products that should be taken (without any side effects whatsoever) before, during and after pregnancy and safe delivery to promote future smooth, safe and healthy child delivery process. The ante natal sessions being done in the hospitals is nice but it is very obvious that it is not adequate, because if it is adequate the rampant cases of difficult child deliveries being recorded these days will not be the case.

For the benefit of my readers, anyone who wishes to take advantage of a more reliable solution to safe pregnancy and smooth child delivery without complications may contact the author of this book for counsel. See the end of this book for my contact address.

WAY TO GOOD HEALTH

I have taken time to study what is necessary to achieve good health and I discovered to my surprise that it does not cost a fortune to achieve good health. Good health is possible especially to anyone who earnestly desires it. It only requires a strong will and determination; it only requires avoiding or refusing eat or do what is not good for your body; it requires you not to put into your body anything that can disrupt the smooth and natural functioning of the body; it requires you to avoid anything that can cause damage to your body cells, organs, tissues, nerves and other things in the body.

The human body can be compared and contrasted with a vehicle (car) which requires certain fluids or components to be in the right places and at the right time for it to function well without any problem. The human body just like a car will function well if you nourish it with the right things in the right quality, quantity and at the right time. If you own a car and fail to put fuel in the tank and put oil instead, if you fail to put water in the radiator and put kerosene instead the car will either to refuse to start or move you to your destination.

But whenever any part of the car is bad or damaged, all you have to do is remove the bad or damaged part and repair it or buy a new part and replace it. But in the case of a human being, you can't remove any part of the body and take it for repair or to even buy an entirely new part for replacement. Therefore, you must make sure at all times to ensure that no part of your body (whether inside or outside of the body) is damaged because you may never get another spare parts to replace it.

It therefore means that if you are a wise human being, you must do everything within your power to ensure that there is no damage of any kind, whether minor or major to any part of your body. You must avoid any damage to your body because prevention is better than cure.

The human body is designed with the ability to be self-sustaining; to be self revitalizing; to be self healing; to be self renewing and you will always be healthy and strong as long as you do not do anything that can disrupt the natural in built mechanism which the creator of the human body has put in place. If you mess around with your body you will be sorry; if you don't protect your body from being invaded by unwanted elements, the end result will be disease, sickness or untimely death.

AIR

Breathing is one of the most basic practices which everybody who desires good health and long life must take very seriously. We take breathing for granted mostly because it is one thing that seem to come naturally to us with little or no effort. When we were born as little babies we just find ourselves breathing. Breathing is one the basic instincts of life which sustains us, we don't learn to breathe, we just start breathing when we are born, but the tragedy is that as soon as we grow older most of us lose the natural or right techniques of breathing properly.

Breathing enables us to take in the necessary prana or life sustaining energies that keep us alive. Breathing the proper way is very vital to good health and long life. The deeper or fuller the breath we inhale into our body the better for our health. We must learn to breathe deeper into the lungs and to exhale the air out of the body in a measured manner. The inhaling and exhaling should not be hurried; it should be a bit slow but according to your capacity; don't breathe too fast or too slow.

Those who are not used to the right pattern of breathing may need to do some practice on a daily basis until they get it right. This can be done in the morning, evening or whenever you can find the time to do so. All you have to do is get a comfortable chair, then sit down, without hunching your back or shoulders. Place your palms flat on top of your laps, your feet flat on the ground and take in a deep breath (let your breath be as deep as possible). Take in a deep breath and breath out in a measured counts of say about 1 to 10, that is, as you breath in start counting from 1 2 3 4 5 until you get to 10 in a fast way within your mind; don't count out loud, just count with your mind. You may decide to count from 1 to 15 or 20 or even more if you can. Just do this regularly everyday, as much as possible. After breathing in and breathing out for a while, you should now breath in and hold the breath (Air) for sometime and count in your mind as usual, that is count from 1 2 3 4 5 until you get to 10 or more if you can, before breathing out the air in your lungs. When you have finished doing the breathing exercises you should say this affirmative words, it doesn't matter whether you believe in God or not, just say it, it will still work for you. Just say these words of appreciation: "thank God for my health that is always very good and will continue to be good." Say this affirmation 4 (four) times at the end of your breathing exercises daily. But if you are sick now keep saying these words until you get well: "thank God for my health that is improving continuously everyday and my health will continue to improve till I regain good health." Say this 4 (four) times at the end of your breathing exercises daily. But take note that as soon as you regain your health and you are no longer sick, you should stop saying these last affirmative words and revert back to saying the first affirmative words earlier given. The first affirmative words is to be said when you are well and not sick but the second one is for when you are sick only, please take note. You can also design your own personal affirmative words if you can and use it everyday after the breathing exercises. If you can design your own personal affirmative words, remember to say them 4 (four) times at the end of the breathing exercises. If you continue to do this on a daily basis with the right attitude and seriousness your breath will gradually begin to adjust for the better and before you know it, you will start breathing properly and your health will start getting a boost. There are other more beneficial breathing exercises that can greatly boost your health no matter how sick you may be. You can find some of these health enhancing exercises in some very good YOGA exercises book or video demonstrations. You can find some of these books or videos in book stores or get them from the internet; you can use Google or any other search engine on the internet to get these very healthy exercises that can make the difference between good vibrant health and a bad one.

Try to find the time to practice deep breathing, you can do this even when you are working, playing or relaxing.

WATER

After prana (fresh Air) energy, the next most vital thing which the human body needs to maintain good vibrant health and long life is WATER. Water is so important that we should never neglect to drink it. Water should be treated with more reverence than even food because the human body can last longer with water than with food. If you were to eat only food without drinking water for some days, you will die quicker in a few days than if you were to drink only water without any food. The body will last far longer with only water than if you were to eat only food without water. Such is the vital importance of water that we should learn to treat water with more respect and importance than many of us do at the moment. Water helps to promote good health and long life. We should always ensure that we not only drink water but the emphasis should be on drinking the right quality, the right quantity and at the right time. It simply means drinking right. If you don't drink right then know that there will be negative consequences to your health. Anyone who cares about good health and long life must take this very seriously. We must be very concerned about where the water we drink is coming from, we must ensure that we drink only the right quality of water. There are many types of water available today. There is rain water, water from the well, borehole water, tap water, river water, packaged water (so called pure water), spring water or rock water, etc.

I always advice that if possible, the only water that we should drink is spring water that has been well processed without using chemicals, but in the absence of spring water then you may drink any other water that has been well processed and free from germs, bacteria, virus, heavy metals, chlorine or any other chemical. It is not advisable to drink water directly sourced from borehole, rain, well, river and others. You may need to buy a very good quality water purifying or distilling system (not water dispenser), where you should first of all put any water you want to drink for processing before collecting the water for drinking.

After getting the right quality of water, you should also ensure that you drink about 8 glasses of water or about 3 liters of water everyday to ensure adequate hydration of the body. There is need to try as much as possible to drink this quantity of water everyday but if you are not used to drinking this quantity of water then you must start learning to drink at least up to 6 glasses or 2 liters of water everyday until you are able to increase the quantity over time. There is need to drink the right quantity of water everyday so that the quantity of water lost from the body as a result of urinating, excreting, sweating, talking or speaking. There is need to replenish all water lost from the body on a daily basis to ensure your good vibrant health. Do not wait until you are thirsty before drinking water, just keep on drinking some small quantity of water every one or two hours until you are able to drink the minimum quantity of water (2 or 3 litres or more) everyday.

The practice of boiling water before drinking should be discouraged because if you boil the water you will end up drinking a dead water with little benefit to your body. If you boil water before drinking you will not only kill the germs or bacteria, you will also destroy most of the beneficial nourishment contained in the water. You should be aware that water has its own natural nourishment which it gives to the body whenever you drink it. The practice of drinking boiled water can deny your body of the right quality of water needed for good health and long life.

Another very important fact which must be taken seriously by everyone who cares about good health and long life is to avoid being thirsty before drinking water. Many people tend to drink water only when they feel thirsty. Drinking water only when you feel thirsty is a very dangerous practice which can affect your health adversely. Always drink at least 2 to 3 liters of water everyday whether you are thirty or not. Your body need water to function properly, therefore you should not wait until you are very thirsty before drinking water; you can make it a point of duty to drink water every one or two hours until you reach the minimum quantity you want to take for the day. Some people avoid drinking enough water just because they want to avoid going to the toilet frequently to urinate or stool. The point is that whether you like it or not, you must urinate and stool because it is part of the metabolic system of the human body designed by the maker of the human body to remove waste products from the body to make it healthy. If you fail to remove waste products from the body as frequently as possible, your health may suffer a set back. So, make sure you drink water whenever you are thirsty and not something else; not juice, milk, beer, mineral (soft drinks) or anything else; whenever you are thirsty just drink at least two or three glass of water immediately before drinking any other thing if you want. The best thing to drink is clean, pure and uncontaminated WATER any other drink is secondary. If you really care about good health and long life then, you should drink mostly water, more than any other drink; drinking fruit juice, milk and other drinks is good but they are not a substitute for water. Avoid any other type of drink as much as possible in favour of water because you body will accept water more than anything else. In fact, the body will sometimes reject any other drink and channel most of it away unused if you give it any other thing when it is highly dehydrated and in dire need of water. A word is enough for the wise.

I have discovered some very good and reliable mineral water processing system which I will not hesitate to recommend to anyone of my readers who may wish to have or acquire one for his or her family use, but it may not be proper to talk about it here because of the fact that there is constant advancement in science and technology which might see the production of a better quality water processing system as times goes on. I can only say for now that for the benefit of my readers who may want me to recommend a good one for them, to such people , I will advice them to contact me through my telephone number or email address as shown at the end of this book so that I can properly advise them on the latest or the most reliable water treatment or processing system at the moment.

FOOD

The importance of food for the maintenance of good health and long life cannot be over emphasized . We already know what will happen to us if we don't eat food but what most people don't know is the quality, quantity and the right time to consume them. Many people eat just for the sake of eating without minding the quality of what they eat. Many people eat food and other things that contribute little or nothing to their health and general well being. The need for a balanced diet is of overwhelming importance for our good health and to promote long life. We should always find out the nutritional contents or value of any food before consuming them so that we don't end up wasting our hard earned money on junk foods and eating what is not good for our health.

When eating food the emphasis should not be to over fill the stomach with too much food; we should eat moderately. Try to drink some little water (not too much) at some intervals when eating your meals or drink some little water at the end of your meal.

Avoid fried food as much as possible; consume mostly cooked food without too much oil and always use good quality oil that promotes good health. Try as much as possible to cook and consume your food without allowing leftovers till the next day if you can afford to be doing this; cook just what you know you can consume for that day only and not more. Food is really beneficial to the body when it is fresh than when it is allowed to stay longer than necessary before eating them. Don't put too much salt in your food, especially after it has been cooked and served. In fact it is better for you not to put any table salt into your food after cooking it; try to put salt into the food during the cooking time and not after cooking. Your health may be put at risk if you fail to adhere to this simple counsel.

Try to avoid food prepared or cooked in an unhygienic and dirty looking environment as well as eating your food in such and environment. Avoid contaminated food; if possible eat only food prepared by you or a trusted person whose sense of hygiene is impeccable. If you must eat with your bare hands make sure you wash your hands very well before eating. And if you are one of those people who like eating frequently with bare hands, always ensure that you cut your fingernails regularly to avoid a situation where dirty or filthy substances containing germs, bacteria and other harmful organisms can hide inside your dirty fingernails, to prevent them from finding their way into your body when eating with your bare hands. Eating the right quality food, eating the right quantity of food and eating the food at the right time is very vital for the promotion of good health and long life. Therefore, knowing what to eat is very crucial and I will advice that wherever you find yourself anywhere in the world try as much as possible to consult a good nutritionist who has a very good knowledge of the types or quality of foodstuffs available in the area where you live so that you can be well advised on the right kind of food that you should be eating to adequately nourish your body so as to provide your body the balanced diet you need to promote good health and long life.

FRUITS AND VEGETABLES

The consumption of fruits and vegetables is the ultimate when it comes to considering what to eat. Fruits and vegetables should be given a priority when considering food consumption issues. I think fruits and vegetables should be eaten more than other food items because they are more acceptable or more useful to the body than other types of food. It is important to check around the environment where you live with a view to finding out the types of fruits and vegetable that are easily available and make a habit of consuming them as much as possible, especially during the season or time of the year when they are more in abundance and if possible try to process them into juice extracts or preserved in a way which can be stored for use when their season of plenty had long gone.

You should always save enough money to buy fruits and vegetables because they are more important in keeping you in good health than most of the other things you eat everyday. Eating different kinds of fruits and vegetables in good quantities will not only provide adequate nourishments for your body but will also help to build up your immune system to a very formidable extent where many sickness or diseases will not be able to invade or survive in any part of your body. It is very important to develop the habit of eating as many types of fruits and vegetables as possible, especially, those type that are not so sweet in terms of their taste; many of these fruits and vegetables which are not sweet and the ones that are bitter or sour in taste are very medicinal and good for the body, they should be eaten as much as possible.

For the benefit of those people who will not be able to get the right varieties of fruits and vegetables that they need for good health, I recommend that they use some good herbal supplement or complements made exclusively with plants, herbs, fruits and vegetable of very high quality to compliment their consumption of fruits and vegetables. Many people do not eat enough quantity and enough quality variety of plants, herbs, fruits and vegetables to provide their body with the required daily minimum needs that is essential to promote good health and long life. I have done some research on some very good plants, herbs, fruits and vegetable supplements extracted from natural plants, fresh fruits and vegetable which I can recommend to anyone who may request me to do so, just get in touch with me through the phone number or email address stated at the end of this book if you are interested.

It is more beneficial to eat or consume fruits when you are hungry and try to eat them at least about one or two hours before you eat your food.

FASTING

Fasting is one very good practice which many people are not taking seriously. Fasting is very good for you; it helps to rid your body of many unwanted elements, acidic substances and some other radical elements that may have sneaked their way into your body. Fasting helps to give the digestive system of the body an opportunity to rest or relax, it is a very wise and sensible thing to do; this allow the body digestive process to go on holiday for a time and no matter how short the holiday the entire body will benefit from the fasting; fasting is a very good practice and you should learn how to fast from time to time because this is one practice that will surely help to promote your good health and put you on the path to long life.

Fasting can be practiced in diverse ways. Total abstainace from food for a few hours to about one, two or three days is a very good practice depending on you ability to bear hunger. For those people who are not used to the practice of fasting, I will advise you not to fast for more than a few hours at a time. You can start by fasting for lets say three, four, five, six or seven hours each day or once a week. You should start with fasting for as many hours as you can each day or each week (may be twice or thrice a week).

You can fast every three days or every four days or every five days or every weekend only. You can decide to fast every two weeks or every three week or once a month. When fasting, do not stay away from food and water longer than your capacity to bear hunger. Do not fast if you are not feeling well enough to do so. If you want to fast for a long period of time, plan for it by eating very well ahead of the chosen date of fasting; eat enough food as much as possible some weeks before the time to put your body in good shape before you commence your fast. When the date of fasting comes try as much as possible to stay away from food for as long as you can before breaking the fast by drinking or eating something. Break your fast with a glass of water or two. You can also break your fast with fruits before eating solid food. You can break your fast by drinking a glass of water and after about 5 to 10 minutes eat some fruits then after another 10 or 20 or 30 minutes you can eat your food.

You may decide to undertake total fasting by not eating or drinking anything at all or you may decide to drink only water during the fasting period. You may also decide to eat some fruits after sometime during fasting. You may decide to drink some water and after sometime you eat some fruits during fasting. You should decide on the type of fasting that you want to undertake. But you should realize that of all the type of fasting system, the best is to abstain from food and water completely for as many hours as you possibly can. The main reason behind fasting is to rid your body of as much toxins or free radical as possible, and to also allow your digestive system a period of rest, which is a very sensible thing to do from time to time, so try as much as possible to do a total or complete fasting. Children should be encouraged to fast also to help promote their good health and to teach them the act of fasting from an early age. Children should not be allowed to fast for too long; after at least two or three hours or more, break their fast and give them food to eat. Just get the child to stay as long as possible before giving food and as they grow up you can increase their fasting time to a suitable level.

The importance of fasting can not be over emphasized. Those who fast are more at an advantage compared to those people who do not. But I can assure you that if you imbibe the practice of fasting your health will gradually become vibrant and if you continue to fast from time to time, you will soon discover that your health is improving no matter how bad it had been. If you can follow all the counsels given in this book together with the practice of fasting, you can be sure that you are on the right road to achieving good health and long life.

EXERCISES

The state of fitness and health of most sportsmen and women is a testimony to the fact that exercise really plays an important role in promoting good health. Apart from those sportsmen and women who indulge in drug abuse or doping, they are usually very healthy people.

It is very good to engage in different types of exercise as it helps to reinvigorate or revitalize the body. Exercises don't have to be tedious or strenuous for it to be beneficial to the body. Exercise can be done according to the ability of each and everyone who wants to promote their health to the next level. You should learn to exercise as much as possible. You should find time to study or observe the various types of sports exercises and practice them according to your ability. You don't have to be perfect in applying them; just try to imitate what the experts are doing. Watch CD/DVD video recordings of sportsmen and sportswomen doing their training exercises or you can go to a gym and practice along with others. Go get yourself some good sport wears and canvas, slipons or sneakers shoe and get ready for your exercise. Find time to go to a good gym or go to any field around your area and start doing some exercises like lifting some small weights (weightlifting) and other exercises; go do some skating; go jogging in the fields or look for a safe road or lane and start jogging, don't run fast, just go as fast as you can, the idea is to just lift and shake your body, go as slow or as fast as possible until your body is well accustomed to the exercise after which you can gradually increase your pace. You can go and play football if you can; you can go swimming if you can. Just go out there and play any game you can play or do any type of exercise that you can do. The more you practice the perfect you become. There are some very good and physical "YOGA" exercises which you can learn and practice right there in your living room; try to buy some of these fantastic yoga exercises CD/DVD videos or check the internet (you may use "Google") and watch the experts performing the exercises and practice along with them.

Another good way to exercise the body which many people do not seem to take very seriously is walking. Walking a long distance is a very good exercise. Many car owners do themselves a lot harm by denying themselves the benefit of trekking or walking. They drive their cars all the time to even places where they can easily trek to. Moving your body by walking directly on the ground (especially walking barefoot on the ground) is very good; walking directly on the earth enables you to directly tap the positive vibrations of the earth. The so called modern civilization has robbed the present day man of the benefit of walking barefooted on the ground in preference of wearing shoes. Shoes or slippers are good but you will do yourself a lot of good if you can find time to place you legs directly on the earth from time to time. Since I don't expect you to be walking about with barefoot, I suggest that whenever you are within your compound premises, try to remove your shoes or slippers and move around when sweeping the compound or planting something in your garden (farm) or even washing your car or doing anything you may want to do. And of course, when you have finished what you want to do, you should wash your legs very well before entering the house. Please remember to ensure that the ground is free from all harmful objects like nails, broken bottles and other harmful things before you walk on the ground without your shoes or slippers.

If you don't like the idea of walking barefoot on the ground then find time (especially on weekends) to walk around your environment from time to time as a form of exercise. Don't always drive your car, you should find time to walk to your destination (not too far) sometimes. You should learn how to walk properly by not hunching your back while walking, instead you should chest your entire rib cage out a little and raise your head or face a bit high as if you are looking at something at the top of somebody's head, this body posture will help you carry your body frame well when walking. Even if you are not going to anywhere in particular, you should find time to move around your neighborhood; just put on some casual dresses or put on your sports wears and stroll around for some good distance and when you are tired of moving around return back home, take your bath, eat something and relax or have your sleep.

Many people sit at home all day doing nothing. No matter how old you are try to keep yourself busy doing something. Many people think that it is demeaning or degrading to do some menial task like sweeping the floor, mopping the floor, cleaning the house, cutting and clearing the grasses in the compound, washing the car, washing the plates, cloths and other house work. When you move around the house doing one form of task or another, you are engaging your body in exercise. Don't sit idle like a piece of furniture in the house, make yourself useful by helping the house helps or those who usually do the house work and do some work exercise; you can tell the house help to go on some break or leave work for sometime to enable you do some of their task instead of sitting in one place all the time, do some exercise that will impact on your health positively.

One very good exercise that most people don't seem to recognize is "DANCING"; dancing is one of the most effective exercises which everyone can do whether you are young or old; dancing is a very good type of exercise which everybody should try to practice as much as possible. I think everyone knows how to dance in one way or another. Dancing can be done any how, all you have to do is shake your body along with your favorite music. Just dance as vigorously as possible for quite sometime and before you know it, you would have done a good exercise and your health will be better for it. Dance as much as possible when you have the opportunity; you don't have to wait until there is a party somewhere before you dance; you can create the opportunity to do your dance exercise right in your living room, just get a good music player, get your favorite music and get going and before you know it, you may have sweated enough and that is good. Do yourself a lot of good by dancing, dance and dance until you get enough exercise from it. You can even dance while in the bathroom, all you have to do is put on your music and keep dancing as you take your bath. If you can't put on your music then sing or mime or hum your favorite music or song and dance on. You can even dance while in the kitchen cooking; you can even dance gently on your office chair though not too vigorously. When you exercise your body regularly you are rejuvenating your body and creating the enabling environment for your continuous good health and long life.   Always remember that dancing is another form of exercise and it is very good for you.

AVOID STRESS

Stress is one subject that is gradually eating deeply into the lives of many people today. The state of many things today, such as the decline of the standard of living for instance is an issue that create so much tension in the mind of many people right now. The economy is not doing as well as many people expect and since the economy of modern man is directly tied to money, the amount of money at the disposal of many people today is on the decline and many people are really stressed up because of their inability to meet their welfare needs and that of other members of their family. Where there is uncertainty in the lives of people they tend to be very highly stressed up; when business is not going on well people tend to be tensed up and this can lead to severe stress that can adversely affect their health.

When things are not progressing the way we want we tend to express negative emotions such as anxiety, worry, irritability, depression, anger, frustration, etc, and this affect our health negatively; whenever we feel threatened in any way we are stressed up and if not well handled our health will begin to suffer.

Whatever the condition we find ourselves we must be careful not to let or allow ourselves to be so stressed to the level where it leads to a health problem, because doing so is a double jeopardy. No matter how bad things may be, we must learn to ease up or free up our minds; we should think of doing things that will put us in a good state of mind. You can go play some games, go to the swimming pool to swim and have fun, go to the beach, go do some other exercise, go watch films or go for any form of entertainment that you enjoy, go chat up with some friends, watch comedy movies, films and other television programmes, just do something to occupy your mind, don't go worrying and sorrowing; don't allow yourself to be overwhelmed by any sad situation you find yourself; try to take life easy and you will begin to fill better with time. Avoid anger and hateful thoughts against your neighbor or your so called enemies because such vengeful hate tends to cloud your mind and aura with negative energies that can back fire against you if not discarded with time. All vengeance should be left for

God to deal with because every action of man must be rewarded when the right time comes. When you avoid the thoughts and actions of harming others whether physically or spiritually, you do yourself a lot of good; you save yourself from guilty or regretful thoughts that could gradually work against your health. When your mind is happy and free, your health will be positively affected also. Many people contemplate suicide when faced with very difficult situations in life, this should not be. No matter how terrible the situation you find yourself, suicide is not an option; no condition is permanent; you can be down today and that does not signify the end of your life. You can still get up tomorrow or anytime in the future. Just keep on keeping on, when there is life there is always hope. If you must die, then don't be the one to cause it, let nature take its course and not you killing yourself by committing suicide. If things are so hard for you and you cannot solve the problem by yourself why not seek help from other people. You can seek help from family members, friends or even from a total stranger. There is nothing bad at all seeking help when you can't help yourself. Who said it must be you only that must solve all your life problems? If you have a serious problem why can't you seek help from God or from someone else? There is no shame or nothing derogatory about seeking for help. God might just use someone to help you out of your problem, so go out there and seek help from every available place if you are stranded instead of committing "SUICIDE", because there is always a way when there seems to be no way.   According to a great man of God (Archbishop Sir George King of the Aetherius Church) whom I respect so much, **"When there is a will there is a way!"**   Be determined to live life to the last moment and one day you may be surprised to see yourself making it in a bigger way.

SLEEP AND REST.

The importance of sleeping and resting adequately can not be over emphasized. Everybody needs adequate sleep to enable them rest and give their body a break. After a hard days work or activity there is need to create time for a good sleep. Finding a quiet place to sleep and rest is very important so as not to be distracted. Taking a good bath before sleeping is a good idea to help sooth the body and prepare it for a nice rest. If you are not in a hurry to sleep off immediately you may need to play some very soft soothing type of music to help relax your mind, but before sleeping off, I think you should put of the music and switch of the power source of the music player. You might also need to put on a dim coloured light, and you may also switch of the light before finally sleeping off if you don't mind. Taking a glass of wine or a bottle of beer sometimes may not be a bad idea if you are finding it difficult to sleep of straight away. I sometimes personally prefer some whiskey, brandy or any available alcoholic drink to relax my mind if I am finding it difficult to sleep, but this practice should not be over done; this should not be turned into a drinking festival, just a little quantity or something reasonable will do. Try as much as possible to get about 7 to 8 hours of sleep everyday.

LAUGHTER/SMILE

Laughter is good for you and you should try to laugh as much as possible. Think of funny jokes, funny things, remember some jokes or anything funny which you have enjoyed before. Try to smile, even if you are alone and believe that no matter how things are at the moment, that it is just a temporary situation and that things will certainly get better, have a positive hope in a better tomorrow. The act of smiling and laughing has a very positive effect on the body and this promotes good health. Always try to be cheerful, always try to feel good and happy even if you are not in a good mood, just imagine it, just pretend that you are very fine and that all is going to be well. Have a very strong faith or belief that no matter how bad and rough things are right now, believe that as long as there is life, that there is hope. For those who are bible believers this counsel in the book of proverbs will go a long way to help you out (Proverbs 17: 22). You don't have to be a Christian to read up that counsel in proverbs and benefit from it. A wise person should always learn good things from anywhere it is available, it should not matter whether it is part of our culture, belief or religious ideology or not. Be confident that there is always a way; believe that there is always a way out of any problem. Realize that any problem is almost half solved if the root cause of the problem can be identified. So try to focus more on identifying the root cause of your problems and devise a way of solving them instead of spending most of your time in a dejected state of mind or stress and strongly believe deep down in your mind that one day the solution to the problem will come.

Listen to good music as much as possible. Get your favorite music collection and play them always, especially when you are stressed up. In fact you should spend some good money to buy for yourself a good music playing set or equipment. Spend some money to buy a lot of music cassettes or CD/DVD disc ; get a good musical collection and store them well away from easy reach of others who may just come and take them away, keep them in good condition and replace anyone that is bad. You should buy all types of music, no matter the language used in singing the music. You can connect with all types of music; buy any music that inspire or excites you. Buy any music with the rights beats, rhythm, melody, lyrics and other features that strikes or make you feel good. Music is a universal language and you can flow along with any music that blends with your soul. Music is a food for the soul and when you can really get the right music for your soul, then stress and other types of life worries can be made to disappear for the moment when the joy of music hits your mind.

DISCIPLINE AND ABSTEINANCE

Many people live their lives in a manner that can be best described a "RECKLESS". So many people have no rule by which they regulate how they live; they just live by doing whatever they feel is comfortable for them. Some just do what they see others do without finding out for themselves whether what they are mimicking or imitating is good for them or not. Because somebody did something or is doing something is not a reason why you should also be doing such a thing; what is good for me might not be good for you.

A person might drink water directly from a water well or river and may not be afflicted by any infection or disease, but someone else might drink that same water and fall very sick after some days. Someone may buy and eat a contaminated food from a road side canteen situated in a very dirty or unhygienic environment and may not be affected or fall sick but some other people may be affected or fall sick due to contamination. This can be so because we all do not have the same level of disease or sickness resistance due to the fact that our immune system are not exactly active on the same level or capacity. Those with a stronger immune system may get away with some unhealthy practices unlike someone else with a weaker or dying immune system. When we are still very young and very active our immune system is usually much stronger than when we start getting old; as we grow old from year to year, our naturally endowed immune system begins to depreciate with time; the situation becomes much worse especially for those people who don't take very good care of their health or it becomes even more dangerous for those who do not observe any health rules or practice that helps to protect, promote and enhance their health.

For you to achieve good health and long life, you must discipline yourself and adopt some health enhancing rules and regulation which can impact positively on your health; there are certain things you cannot do and there are others you should be doing to create the right conditions for you to be healthy. There are many health hazards which you should be aware of; just as there are many health promoting code of conduct which can go a long way in ensuring that you continue to remain healthy; so that you don't slide from good health to bad health. For instance we all know that it is a good thing to take our bath three times or two times everyday but how many people are able to observe this strictly? How many people do take their baths and use a good body sponge to scrub their bodies very well when taking their baths at least five times a week? How many people know the benefit of using or putting some disinfectants into their water before using it to take their baths about four or five times a week? How many people know the right way to brush their teeth by moving the toothbrush up and down or from the top of the teeth to bottom of the teeth instead of just brushing haphazardly? How many people do find time to scrub their tongues with a spoon or anything that can effectively scrub the tongue without causing any injury? Scrubbing the tongue helps to remove some thick substances which are usually trapped within the towel of the tongue; scrubbing your tongues at least once or twice a week before using your toothbrush on your teeth and tongue is good for your mouth health.

How many people do take their time to chew their food very well before swallowing them? Do you know that your health might be endangered if you are not chewing your food very well before allowing them into your body system? Do you also know that it is wise to eat your last food of the day at least between 5-7 pm everyday, so that your food can start digesting before you go to bed for your sleep? Do you know it is good to maintain a fixed eating time for your three or two square meals everyday so that your body can know when to expect food and start processing them for your good health everyday? Do you also know that it is not wise to eat anyhow in between your fixed time of feeding everyday?

How many people really take their time to wash their hands thoroughly before eating with bare hands?

If you live in a mosquito infested area why not take proactive measures to prevent mosquitoes from invading your house by installing mosquito nets on your doors, windows and other open spaces to prevent mosquitoes from gaining entry into your living room/bedrooms?

Why not use a mosquito net to cover yourself before sleeping everyday? Why not take steps to do away with the pool of water near your house to prevent mosquitoes from breeding more armies of deadly mosquitoes that might end up terrorizing you and your family members or households on a daily basis?

Do you know that the quality or type of mattress or foam you sleep on everyday can make you sick or create pains all over your body and affect your health adversely? Why sleep on just anything and not on a good quality mattress (foam)?

Why sit on just any type of unsuitable and uncomfortable chair that can create neck, back, waist or general body pains when there are good quality chairs that will ensure that your body is well positioned when seated to avoid body pains? Anyone who spend a lot of time sitting behind a desk whether at home or in the office, certainly need to use a very good quality office chair and table. The acquisition of good quality office chairs (especially the rotating type) should be taken very seriously by all employers of labour to protect their employees from the health consequences associated with sitting on a bad quality chair and desk. In fact I will advice all workers or employees who take their health seriously to save enough money from their salaries to enable them buy for themselves a very good quality chair for office use to protect themselves from the health implications of always sitting on a bad quality chair. If your employer refuses to reimburse you after spending your money to buy a good quality chair for office use, you can simply take away your chair when leaving for another job elsewhere if you get another job in future.

I strongly advice anyone who is interested in good health and long life to make the necessary effort or sacrifice to save or even borrow (get a loan) to buy a very good quality mattress (foam) for sleeping and to also acquire a very good quality office chair because their continuous good health might depend on this. I find it very amusing seeing many people saving or borrowing a lot of money to buy things that are very unnecessary when compared to their health. I consider people who prefer to invest a lot of money in other things without first of all investing in things that can promote their good health and long life as people with misplaced priority. I regard persons who don't consciously invest in their health as either foolish or ignorant. No amount of money can be too much for buying things like food, health products, furniture, medicine or anything that you need to achieve good health and long life. Do I need to still emphasize here that it is only those people who are alive and in good health that can enjoy the things of this world. Spending whatever amount of money on anything else without first spending on things that can keep you alive to enjoy other worldly things sounds very foolish and illogical; it will make more sense for you to buy the things you need to keep your good health in good shape and intact. Therefore if it makes sense to spend your money on things that promotes good health and long life, then I guess it will also make sense for you not to spend your money in buying things that will either disrupt or terminate your good health. Many people use their own hard earned money to buy things that will either make them sick or make them start dying gradually.

Why use your money to buy cigarettes, alcoholic drinks, junk foods, hard drugs like cocaine, heroine, marijuana, and others that might disrupt or interfere with your health? Why buy and consume too much sugar loaded food or drinks, unhealthy cooking oil, expired or contaminated foods or drinks, as well as other consumables which is not good for your health? Always watch your body for any sign of ill health or discomfort, if you notice any consistent discomfort, don't hesitate to see a medical doctor or any qualified alternative or complementary medical/health practitioner for advice. I want to assure you that if you follow the simple counsel given in this book about how to achieve good health and long life seriously enough from a very young age, you may never fall sick again for the rest of your life. If you start practicing these counsels when you are already advanced in age you will notice a vast improvement of your health on a continuous basis until you achieve good stable healthy condition. I am also indicating here that if you find out that you are always sick even after following the counsel in this book for a minimum of five to seven years of serious practice, then I will suggest you see a qualified spiritualist or a powerful prophet or man of God for healing because your health problem might be a spiritual attack and not ordinary sickness.

Consuming foods, fruits, vegetables and drinks moderately is better than consuming them excessively, there is need to balance your consumption of the things you eat so that you don't end up eating too much or too little of everything you need to be healthy. It is your responsibility to always ensure that you buy or consume only the things that can enhance your health and stay away from those things that has the capacity to jeopardize your health. Try as much as possible to eat only foods that will provide your body with proteins, vitamins, minerals and other nourishments that your body need for good health. Eat food that is rich in fibers to help your digestive and waste elimination process and also reduce the eating of meats and starchy foods. Try to keep a moderate weight, don't get too fat or too slim, if possible go and see those who can help you check your body mass or index and try to keep it right. It is very important to make sure that you make enquiries about the health benefit of any food, drink or anything before buying or consuming them; you need to ask questions or investigate the health or nutritional value and benefits of any consumable item before allowing them into your body. Always remember that your body does not have a duplicate, so do everything possible to preserve it in good health to enable you live long.

Authors contact address:

Phone number: +234 08030892274   or 08030892274

Email address: clembeam2060@yahoo.co.uk